SPONTANEOUS KUNDALINI AWAKENINGS

Healing the Damage Through IFS

PETER LEGÅRD NIELSEN

SPONTANEOUS KUNDALINI AWAKENINGS

Healing the Damage Through IFS

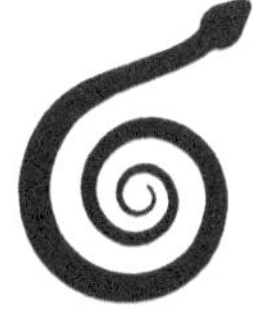

Foreword by Robert Falconer,
the author of 'The Others Within Us'

CONTENT

FOREWORD

This book is a delight. Peter Legård Nielsen is a well-known novelist in Denmark. It is so refreshing to have a psychology book written by a sensitive writer. Many psychotherapy books are written so poorly they are almost painful to read even though their content is very valuable. The diagnostic and statistical manual, which is the Bible for psychotherapy in America, is an example of hideous tortured prose and ugly pompous neologisms. The subject matter of this book fascinates me but it would be a good read even if you weren't especially interested in this area. Even for the people with the most experience working with Kundalini Peters methods will add something new. His deep understanding of IFS gives him a unique framework to do this work. He has created an original, dialogical-relational way of working with this ancient dynamic. I am hoping that Peter will give us many more books in English on psychology and spirituality.

This specific work on Kundalini energy is fascinating and it makes a great example of a more general point. There are many forms of psychological experience that in the modern West we hold as illness that actually can have great value. Peter quotes Carl Jung on this. "What was normally perceived as a pathological state could actually be understood as a very meaningful symbolic process through which the clients became healthier." Studies of the intersection between psychosis and spirituality, for example those of the psychologist Isabel Clarke in England, or the anthropologist Tanya Luhrmann in America, support this important conclusion. Culturally we do not have good containers in which to receive non-ordinary experiences. Hearing voices, for example, was considered a sign of psychosis until very recently. This despite the fact that in couples who had lived together 45 years or more when one partner had died 80% of the survivors heard their voice. So hearing voices is obviously not always pathological. Under certain circumstances it's normal. Also, Socrates, often considered the origin of Western rational philosophy, heard voices his entire life. Until very recently, and still in many quarters, if a psychotherapist encourages a client to dialogue with the voices they hear it is considered malpractice. There are many other areas where non-ordinary experience and spiritual experience are pathologized. This book gives a strong clear example of how dealing with one of these areas, Kundalini energy, in a non-pathologizing way is beneficial.

Some skeptical readers will be tempted to dismiss the entire area of Kundalini energy as some New Age fantasy. I believe the descriptions of Kundalini express an underlying reality, a basic bio-psychological experience that happens to many humans. This introduction is not the place for an extended exposition of this belief but I want to call attention to one important example that might open even the most skeptical mind. The San and the Kung people, often referred to as bushmen of the Kalahari, report very similar experiences which are recognized and honored in their culture. These people have had no contact with the cultures of India where ideas of Kundalini come from. The main religious and healing ceremonies of the San are all-night ritual dances. In these dances the first goal is to stimulate the sacred energy, num, which lives dormant at the base of the spine. They heat this energy by their dance until it boils and comes up through their spine. When it has done this, they go around and heal others with their hands. Many people including Richard Katz and Bradford Keeney have written extensively about this so we are not reliant on only one source.

Another point which may give pause to the skeptical reader is talking with parts of the person and to the Kundalini energy itself. In Internal Family Systems therapy we encourage people to dialogue with their parts all the time so this is not surprising to us or new. Internal Family Systems therapy is one of the fastest growing modalities and there are many records and testimonies as to its effectiveness. So hopefully even the most skeptical of readers might bracket their belief system and acknowledge the possibility that internal dialogue can be very healthy. Peter takes internal dialogue even further than many IFS therapists and he dialogues with the Kundalini energy itself, and with locks or blockages in the person's body. This is a very powerful and effective technique even if it is counter-intuitive for the modern Western mind. To me the personalism of Martin Buber and others provide a rigorous philosophical background for these attitudes. Martin Buber divided all relationships into two categories; I-It relations and I-Thou relations. He clearly stated that we could have I-Thou relationships with anything including a rock. He also stated that I-Thou relations deepen our experience. He indicated that I-It relations are the source of much, or perhaps all, evil. Peter's work is a great example of using I-Thou relationships with the beings who inhabit our inner subjective world.

In the United States there are several psychologists, notably Emma Bragdon, who are working with Kundalini experiences and clearly separate them from psychopathology. Peter's method of working is distinct and I believe an advance on what has been done. In conclusion I want to state that over the years I have referred many difficult clients to Peter. His methods, however innovative and radical they may appear to the reader, work. This is to my mind the real, radically pragmatic way to evaluate psychotherapy; does it relieve human suffering? Peter's work does.

Robert Falconer, councilor, teacher
and author of 'The Others Within Us'
and other books

1

INTRODUCTION

One of the places where explorations in the spiritual field can go terribly wrong is when working with Kundalini energy, traditionally understood as the life force or the sexual energy that is coiled as a serpent at the bottom of the spine in our bodies.

In the Eastern tradition working with the Kundalini energy is supposed to be one of the ways to spiritual enlightenment, but sometimes the process takes an unexpected turn, where it feels like the Kundalini energy is destroying the body and the mind. One of the pitfalls is not having an experienced teacher or guru when entering into this field. In some cases, the process can even start by itself leaving people totally unprepared for what is happening to them.

Individuals who have a spontaneous activation of the Kundalini may experience severe physical and psychic problems for the rest of their lives. There are many examples of this, including literature and on the internet. To make matters worse, the traditional healthcare system has no understanding of what happens during a Kundalini awakening, and perhaps never will. These people have typically been diagnosed with hypochondria, schizophrenia, or psychosis.

I am one of those people who experienced the awakening of the Kundalini energy as a complete destruction of who I was. For many years, I lived with a feeling of being thrown out of my own life. I had to be so controlled to repress the explosive energy that it felt as if life was just a cartoon around me. Everything seemed to be flat and oozed of emptiness.

My disastrous experience with Kundalini took place about forty-five years ago. Since then I have gained some insight into what happened to me. Six years ago, I began integrating a new and experimental psychotherapy called *Internal Family Systems* (IFS) in my work as a therapist. IFS has a strong element of spirituality, paired with shamanistic techniques, and for the first time a therapy seemed to provide me with a key to unlock the unexplainable which took place inside of me all those years ago. One day, I had gained enough courage to confront the Kundalini again.

One day at my clinic, a client came for her IFS session and was very disturbed. She had experienced something really upsetting, and as she talked, I realized she was talking about a Kundalini awakening. I had often wondered if I would be able to help people who had this experience so that they shouldn't go through the same misery I had gone through. While listening to the client I got a clear impression of what I could do to help her, based on my knowledge of this state and my work with IFS.

This book is a description of the work with Kundalini that emerged from this session and later sessions with other clients, and how I found a way to help them. I will issue a warning up front: Therapeutic work should always be taken seriously and practiced responsibly, and that is even more true for this kind of work, because the therapist enters a dangerous field of fear and confusion. The good news is that it can be done; it is indeed possible to tame the Kundalini.

2

MY OWN EXPERIENCE

In 1979, when I was 18, I spent the summer at a small yoga camp. I had just finished high school and would begin my higher education after the summer break. The world was supposed to be open to me, I was expected to have the time of my life, but instead, I felt awful, living in what felt like a desert devoid of possibilities. During high school, I lost connection with my friends from elementary school. The high school was 45 minutes away by bus from the village where I grew up, and since my classmates and I never had any time to socialize after school, I never really got the chance to connect with them. Most of them lived close to each other, and on Mondays, I could only sit and listen to all the stories of what had happened during the weekends, the parties that they had been to, and who had hung out with whom.

Over the years I have read many descriptions

and heard many people talk about how wonderful it is to live in a small village, where the inhabitants know each other and help each other out, where there is community. Each time I have wondered if the writer or the speaker has actually tried to live in such a small village, or if it was more a romantic idea emerging from visits to such places. If the locals don't think that you belong there, living in a small village can be brutal and isolating. I felt very ostracized in the village where I grew up, and this added to the feeling of loneliness that I experienced in high school. In the end, I felt that I knew no one.

In addition to that, my father was dying. Actually, he had been dying for years, and everything in the house revolved around his health. Each time I walked through the door, I felt as if I had stepped into The House of Death. I had to protect my father from my mother's anger about him being ill. I had the sense that I was the only responsible person there, taking care of the family, while at the same time I was very sad for my dad and could understand my mother's fear-ridden anger.

A couple of years earlier, a woman who worked at the library and wasn't a local, had noticed my loneliness when I borrowed books. She took a weekly yoga class and asked if I wanted to come along and check it out. We continued taking classes together for two seasons, and I enjoyed her company as we drove back and forth in her car. Then she decided to stop, because she was busy with other things, and I lost contact with her, but I continued to go to the yoga classes. I found them interesting, and they gave me something to do outside the house one evening every week.

Some days into this hot, desert-like vacation, I got a phone call that really surprised me. It was from the woman who taught the yoga classes. I already knew that she was aware of my interest in the *asanas*. Now she told me she was having a summer camp and that there was an empty space she wanted to offer to me. As a family, we didn't have a surplus to spend on unnecessary items, so my first question was the price. The woman, let's call her Sara, said that instead of paying I could help her and her husband with practical things during the training. I was happy to say yes and even had a vague feeling of being chosen.

Sara and her husband were also recent arrivals and lived in a former farmhouse on the outskirts of the village. Even though this was something we had in common, I still felt like a stranger with them, but for different reasons than with the local villagers. I was shy and wasn't knowledgeable about all the kinds of mysticism that they were studying. I knew nothing about Jung, whom they were fond of and often cited, especially (as with other new age movements) his theory about synchronicity. And they came from the big city.

Over the next few days, I got to know the other participants who, in many ways, seemed exactly like Sara and her husband. I often felt like the local fool. I had no experience with things like tantra or *cosmic orgasm*, which were talked about in conversations that I eavesdropped on at the beach in the sparkling sun. During dinner at the big table in the farmhouse, I listened to conversations about how certain vegetables to some of the participants tasted exactly like chicken. I felt slightly ashamed of the fact that I would probably have preferred a slab of red meat to the porridge served at most meals.

For many hours a day, we did yoga and tai chi exercises and practiced meditation for long periods of time. This was new to me, as we had only briefly meditated at the beginning and end of the weekly yoga classes.

Returning to The House of Death when the camp ended was depressing. After spending an extended period of time with all these people, loneliness crept over my skin as I walked through the door. It was devastating and felt like running into a brick wall. After that, the summer seemed endless. I was eager to start my new education, in a city far away where I would once again have to ride the bus for hours back and forth.

One day while I was practicing the meditation that I had learned, I had a sensation, like a very thin veil falling to the floor of the inner world that I was seeing in front of my eyes. It was subtle, like a gentle breeze.

In bed that evening, I found to my surprise that I was unable to fall asleep. I added it up to the feeling of being in this vacant, lonely world. It was the weekend, and I had biked to the beach to sunbathe in the dunes and swim in the waves, but besides that, I had spent most of my time reading. I was probably not tired.

At the same time, I felt a certain nervousness that surprised me, like something was going on inside of me, yet I didn't know what it was. As in meditation, I had an inner vision of vague pictures. When morning came, I hadn't slept at all.

The next night I still couldn't sleep. I started to get worried. A strange nervousness had invaded me and made it even harder to fall asleep. Somehow I felt that the nervousness was connected to the images I saw while meditating.

In the following days, it became increasingly

weirder. I started having strange energy movements up my spine. It was like a burning feeling in my nerves, and I experienced a strong, almost violent pressure on my skull, coming from below. When I closed my eyes, the images took over. As the days without sleep passed by, they became more and more violent and terrorizing. It seemed like I was brought back to a medieval world, probably the Inquisition, where brutal, muscular men with leather caps over their heads, naked, sweating torsos, wielding chains and axes in their hands, performed unspeakable violent acts to chained-up women. It was worse than any horror movie I had ever seen. If I stayed too long with the visions, they took over completely and infused my nervous system with a terrifying fear that made my teeth clatter and my body shake. I had lost the ability to sleep. Each time I tried to find sleep, I got lost and instead ended up in endless meditation. It seemed to lay above sleep, blocking my access to it.

I didn't dare to tell my parents about what was happening. Our big concern was my father's health, and I wouldn't want to take the attention away from that, especially not as I was supposed to be the one in control. I also knew that if I told them about what had happened, my parents wouldn't be supportive, but rather concerned with what I might have done wrong and what the neighbors might think. My worst fear was that I was going mad and would have to be locked up in a mental institution. *Paranoid schizophrenia* were the words I heard over and over again in my anxious mind. I was so used to taking care of myself that I didn't reach out to anybody. And I was hyper vigilant to be in control. In daylight, I was so much in control that no one ever noticed what was going on.

As the days progressed, I became more and more afraid of going to bed and be confronted with the terrifying torture scenes, but then the disturbing images started to appear before my eyes in pure daylight. I had to stop fixating on objects for a longer period of time and let my eyes jump from place to place, like small birds, to keep them away.

Finally, my fear made me contact Sara. I had discovered that driving was one of the activities that helped me the most, because it commanded my attention, especially if I drove fast. When I arrived at the remote farm, she was unfortunately not at home, only her husband, who always made me feel rather shy and slightly uncomfortable. I told him what had happened but, much to my surprise, he didn't seem to understand what I was trying to put into words. Actually, it seems like he was envious of what I was going through. For him, it was a breakthrough, for me it had become a question of life and death; my mental health was at stake.

He had one piece of advice for me and that was to get grounded. When I asked him how I should do this, he told me to go into the garden at home, dig a hole, and stand in it with bare feet. And then what, I asked? Then you will be able to connect with the earth, he answered. I had a strange desire to laugh aloud. This technique seemed like much too little and much too late, compared to the forces fighting inside of me.

That night, as my parents were asleep, I went into the garden and dug the hole. I stood on the cold ground for fifteen minutes, but nothing happened. I decided to stay there longer and wondered if I had done something wrong. Should I have spread the pile of dirt that I had dug up, on my feet? Finally, I gave up. I didn't feel more grounded than when I started, and that night the vision once again increased in intensity.

My eyes were burning with tiredness and my body was sore from lack of sleep, but I still had this intense, unstoppable pressure of energy shooting through my spine to my head.

One day, as I was sitting in my room, I lifted my gaze and saw something that made me gasp in terror. It was as if I perceived reality as it really was when it was not mediated by our senses. Everything around me, the furniture, the walls, the plants in the window, the books in my bookcase, and the chair I was sitting in, consisted of vibrating atoms. I was just a rhythm in space, with a certain density that made me different from the other things in space. But it also felt like I might vibrate into a thousand pieces anytime. There was no solid core. I had no clue what held me together.

Two days later, after a long sleepless week, I decided to drive out to Sara once again, hoping to meet her, and this time I was lucky. She was much more compassionate than her husband, but in the end, I had the same feeling that she was actually envious of what had happened to me. She called a healer she knew, but he was busy and had no time to see me. Finally, she gave me the advice to go to bed that night and imagine the face of God coming down to me. That always made her go to sleep, she told me.

I was so desperate that I was willing to do anything, even though it didn't sound like it would lead anywhere. That night, I tried to do as she had suggested and imagined God's face in front of me. It felt like he came up from my feet like the bearded God of The Old Testament and hovered over me. It was as if we were inside a shield of blue glass while the terror visions were outside, at a distance that made them somewhat less scary.

Suddenly God's face burst. And what was left felt like dew, tears rolling down my cheeks from my exhausted eyes.

Then I heard a singing tone, like a violin string, sharp, cold, cutting. I knew where it came from and went into the kitchen and opened the drawer with knives. Part of me was totally mesmerized by the shade of the blade of one of the knives. This part wanted to kill itself. As I reached for the knife and grabbed it, other parts of me were immediately activated and stepped in and made me drop the knife. They made me turn around and blaze through the door to my parent's bedroom where I screamed that I had tried to kill myself and that they had to stop me.

My parents woke in total confusion. Seeing their faces as they sat up in the bed, the shame of being suicidal came over me. I knew how devastating it would be for them to have this impossible son.

My father called the doctor, and luckily we were able to see him right away. The clinic wasn't yet open, but it was impossible for me to wait. Also, I didn't dare stay with my parents as they would start asking questions about what had happened. I was so restless that I decided to walk to the clinic while my father got dressed.

On the way to the doctor in this small village, I suddenly realized that I had lost track of where I was. I couldn't find the clinic. After a while, my father drove up beside me in his car, rolled down the window and asked, what had happened, why hadn't I gone straight to the doctor's clinic?

The next surprise came in the doctor's office. After we sat down, I revealed, quite agitatedly, what had happened to me, painstakingly aware that my father was sitting right behind me, listening. When I finished, the doctor said he didn't believe me. He practiced meditation himself and was convinced it could not lead to such problems as I had experienced. I wanted, at any cost, to avoid a diagnosis of mentally ill, and as I sensed that he was headed in that direction, I managed to control myself. I realized that I was alone in this. I just wanted things to go back to the way they were a week ago.

Somehow I succeeded in convincing the doctor that I was no longer suicidal. I think he also wanted to believe that. I might have come across as weird, but I belonged to a well-respected family in the village. I just wanted to get out of his office, go home, and take care of myself, but at the same time, I knew that I needed help to fall asleep. He gave me a prescription for anti-anxiety and sleeping pills and an injection with a sleeping aid. As we left, I didn't dare to look at my father, embarrassingly aware of the public shame I had exposed him to.

Arriving home, sleep finally caught up with me and I collapsed on the bed.

When I woke up, I wasn't sure what had happened. The clock showed almost the same time, as when I had fallen asleep, and I realized twenty-four hours must have passed. Then the events of the last days rolled over me again, like a wave in the sea. I was relieved. I had slept. Now I could return to normal, how things had been a little more than a week ago.

I put my feet on the floor and had the strange sensation that this was not going to happen. First my hands started shaking, then my whole body, and I could barely control the shaking.

I got up and walked into the living room to confront my parents. They were sitting there, waiting for me. I felt deeply ashamed.

As best as I tried, I couldn't hide the state I was in. My body was still shaking. Their worried and mistrusting faces met my gaze. I said I was sorry. Somehow I managed to convince them that I would never again try to kill myself. Then I slid like a shadow out of the room.

That night, I took the sleeping pill and the anti-anxiety pill, and the medication made the images behind my eyelids a little less aggressive, thought they didn't disappear and remained extremely violent. I had spent most of the days walking in the woods. It seemed that walking was the only thing I could do. If I sat still, the thoughts of what had happened started to overwhelm me. I had never heard of anyone who had experienced anything like this. I knew nothing about Kundalini. I thought I was the only person who had had this experience. I was determined not to dissolve into madness.

I still couldn't sleep and laid in bed for hours, trying to relax as the violent images slowly re-emerged. Finally, as morning came, I fell into a light sleep that lasted a couple of hours.

Over the next few days, I began to realize the terrifying scope of what had happened. I couldn't sit still for very long, but had to get up and walk, up and down hills, through forests, over barren fields, and along the coastline. My eyes had changed, and it sometimes seemed like I could see deep into the ground. What I saw was only death, all the death that was underground, corpses, skeletons, maggots, decay.

I also discovered that it was impossible for me to read, as there was so much energy in words, that I got dizzy from the pressure in the head and began shaking when I tried. That really scared me. I had just started my studies a few weeks earlier and was supposed to read a lot but found that I was unable to. Reading had always been my go-to, my comfort, my way to escape, and now I had been forced to give that up as well.

One of the first nights after my suicide attempt I got the idea to turn the architect lamp on my table over the bed so that it would be shining right into my eyes when I lay on my back. Along with the pills, this made the torture images in my mind less intimidating, less visible. I wouldn't have guessed that one could sleep with such a strong light directly into the eyes, but it worked, at least for some hours.

I never knew what mood I would be in when I woke up. Some days I woke up with an extreme surplus of energy and felt like I was in an almost divine flow. On those days I would stop strangers in the street and talk to them and continue a conversation for a long time, something I would previously have been much too shy and inhibited to do.

Other days, I woke up with what felt like a lead helmet on my head and I was deeply depressed. On those days I could hardly speak to other people, but just needed to stay with myself and that heavy weight in my body.

But no one knew. I had my strong will and was used to being extremely controlled, and that worked for me now. The study wasn't that difficult, and I picked up what I needed to know without reading. My parents believed I was well again because that was what I told them, and it was also easier for them to believe. They had no idea about how my nights went.

One day out walking, I started to see our whole society revealed, like I had seen the true nature of reality in my room just days before my breakdown. I saw all the massive pillars that we had built through time to support the basic structure, but I also saw that it was nothing but cardboard. It could easily collapse. Civilization was a fraud, a comfort we allowed ourselves to indulge in, but it wasn't real. Underneath was the rot, the slithering snakes, the glittering slime.

Snakes had become my most persistent companions. I had always been extremely scared of snakes, to the extent that I couldn't even touch a picture of a snake. Now I saw them everywhere when I closed my eyes, and I felt them moving in my body, especially in my spine. I knew this to be an indication of a person going mad.

One day I had so much pressure in my head that, in pure desperation, I sat down and wrote all the words in my head on a piece of paper. It gave me a strange feeling, as if I was slowly pulling a spring out of my brain. When I looked down on the paper, quickly letting my eyes slide over it so as not to get too energized, I realized I had written a complete poem. It was finished, without anything to correct or change. And my head felt light, without pressure. This lasted a couple of hours.

From that experience, I learned to empty my head several times a day by writing a poem describing the images that I saw. If I forgot or didn't have the time, there was a price to pay, but I could always find relief by putting pen to paper.

One of the things that was hard for me to explain to myself, and probably would have been even harder to explain to other people, had I tried, was a feeling of having lost the sense of who I was. My ego was gone or destroyed. What was left was more like waves on the surface of the ocean. In a sense, I could be anything, and yet there was this density, this accumulation of particles, this beam of light inside that was me.

For three years I lived like this. I was able to read again, but sleep was a challenge every night, and I got accustomed to using my architect lamp to make the brutal images harder to see. I was still on an emotional rollercoaster, with good days and bad days, but my will to be perceived as normal was so strong that no one knew anything about this internal struggle.

Some days I was filled with anger at Sara and her husband for leading me into this mess without even a warning and for being unable to help me. I had contacted them one time after my suicide attempt, but during the visit, it became obvious to me that their main focus was *not* getting involved so they couldn't be accused of anything. One day, much to my surprise, a former participant in the first yoga class told me that they were very disappointed in me for having abandoned them. This made it clear to me that they had no idea of what was going on. I never saw them again.

During these first years I also had an experience that became recurrent. Some nights when I had managed to fall asleep I woke up unable to move. I learned that this is what happens to the nervous system when we sleep so that we don't move around. Sleepwalking happens when this mechanism fails. But being awake and lame, without any possibility of moving, was scary. It always happened the same way, a strong current would begin to run through my body, sometimes up from the sacrum and out through the head, and sometimes from the head down into the legs. I couldn't stop it.

Having finished my studies, I decided to move to Peru for a year. I had a perhaps naive feeling that going to a developing country would get me in contact with a simpler way of living that could bring me down to Earth. Also, it was as far away from Denmark as I could get. I wanted to start with a clean slate, a place where no one knew me, and see if I could survive. During the process with the Kundalini, I had lost the fear of dying. It felt like it had already happened, despite my failed suicide attempt.

I found work in Peru as a foreign aid worker in a remote Andean village, and I did succeed in my aim to create a new life. Peru also gave me what turned out to be long-term diseases. I was finished with my body. I felt it had betrayed me in the worst possible manner. I didn't care when I got food poisoning or when I got parasites from living too primitively among peasants in the mountains. I didn't go to the doctor but just lived with it, that is, until I returned to Denmark and realized that many of my symptoms were so far advanced that the doctors couldn't help me and that the pain had become chronic.

I became a writer. When my first novel got published it was, much to my surprise, sold to a book club and printed in thousands of copies. I could thank the awakening of the Kundalini for that career, but it felt like a gift wrapped in poisonous snakes. Internally, I just grew colder and more controlled—more hollow and empty—as the years passed by, haunted by the pains in my body. I felt my body deserved it.

Ten years after my breakdown I decided to go into bioenergetic therapy. I had stayed far away from any kind of yoga and meditation and had also been suspicious of psychotherapy. I allowed no one to mess around with my inner world. The bioenergetic therapist had actually reached out to me, and it took some courage on my part to say yes. Deep down I probably knew that I couldn't go on the way I had done for so many years.

Bioenergetic therapy gave me back my body. I still believe it was the safest path and the only place for me to start therapy. I was too good at being mental. It had always been my survival tool. With the return of my body came a hitherto unknown sensitivity that seemed partly innate, partly from the Kundalini experience. After that, I discovered Rolfing, an advanced body therapy. It was so convincing as a therapy that I soon began training to become a Rolfer myself. During the training, I discovered that I could see inside the body with my hands in ways that most people weren't able to.

When my hands touched the body of the person I was training on, I got a full 3-dimensional picture in my head of the anatomy under the skin. I was also able to feel the trauma in the client on the table, not just the physical, but also the related emotions. Under my hands were the exiles and protectors that IFS talks about. I could sense them and work with them, even if I didn't know that that was what they were called. The Kundalini awakening appeared to have radically opened my senses. I also began to see things that we normally do not speak of, and I couldn't deny that I was able to notice spiritual beings like personal guides, spiritual masters, archetypes, angels and archangels, and also dead people and demons. We were surrounded by them.

Getting my body back also gave me a sense of Self. A calm force inside of me was capable of sensing into other people and understanding their point of view without losing my own. Instead of focusing on polarizations, I became aware of an ever-present third way.

While practicing bioenergetic therapy, I published several novels and earned a living as chairman of The Danish Fiction Writers Association. The job helped me shape my feeling of Self as I needed extremely well-defined boundaries. When

I first took the chairman seat, I didn't realize that some writers were desperate to get acknowledgment and scholarships, and they suddenly saw me as a person of power and were prepared to exploit and sometimes even blackmail me, if they found a weak spot. The Kundalini experience had taught me how to lean into the force of calm, a quality that became especially important in the critical and dramatic negotiations I regularly had with The Ministry of Culture on behalf of the writers. I doubt that I would have been strong enough for the job without the Kundalini experience and the emergence of Self that it created.

Luckily, I had also regained my sense of fear. Living in a world where nothing scares you is like living in a world without values, a bit zombie-like.

During those years I had what I will call four challenges.

The first was *horror vacui*. Since I had started to feel how the Kundalini experience destroyed my ego, I had gotten increasingly afraid of being *nothing*. One day I decided to sit down and allow myself to be exactly that. The terror as I stepped into the field of *nothingness* was overwhelming. But I found the courage to meet it. I allowed it to take me over, and I became *nothing*. The moment I opened my eyes as *nothing*, I expected everything to be changed, but in reality nothing had changed. The world around me looked exactly like before, and inside I felt exactly the same. But the fear of *being nothing* was gone. Without changing anything, a change had taken place.

The next challenge was the fear of the female archetype that many men seem to have. For me, it was mixed with the knowledge that the Kundalini was perceived as female and therefore dangerous.

As with the challenge of *nothingness*, I sat down and contacted the archetype. When she came into my vision I stepped forward to surrender fully to her. The moment it happened was so terrifying that I could feel the hair on my arms and neck stand up. I was afraid of being swallowed, killed, and devoured. The first thing I realized was that the female archetype could actually do that and that men in that sense were right in fearing her. The next thing I realized was that she would never do that, she had no desire to kill men, it was simply not something she would ever do. The fear subsided, and there was trust and harmony between the female archetype and me.

Since then, I have been able to get better along with women; it's as if they sense that I no longer fear them deep down in the primordial depths of my psyche.

The third challenge was to meet the archetype of the snake. At that time I had already learned to be with the snakes that relentlessly slithered through my consciousness and scared me. One day, I stretched out my finger in the inner world and asked a big cobra to bite me with its poison-dripping tooth. It was a moment of terror as I waited for the poison pump through my veins. Then I realized that the snake withdrew a bit and I moved my finger forward. It didn't bite. It wouldn't or couldn't. This taught me a very important lesson, maybe the most crucial in this whole story: *the inner world can't attack me if I'm not afraid of it.* It turned out to be true in all situations and it significantly lowered my level of anxiety. Something relaxed and settled in me in a good way. It also made it much easier for me to be with and work with what we call demons when they showed up in my clients during our sessions. I wish I had known this truth from the beginning.

One day, sitting in deep contact with my inner world, I saw just to the right of me the head of a cobra align with my head. It felt like we were twins in the stream of time. I knew that the snake could be perceived as a representative of the nervous system and I did not fear it any longer. In what seemed like a reckless letting go, I decided in that instant to let my brain melt together with the cobras. It was like being hit by a strong electrical current, like something silently cried out as in Edvard Munch's painting *The Scream*. I saw a picture of my brain and the snake's brain slide together in an electric glow, wobble against each other and finally fall into place, while lightning radiated out in beams. It reminded me of how a spark occurs when the human egg is fertilized and the area around is flooded with zinc. Somehow we merged.

This experience prepared me to face the fourth challenge, to confront the Kundalini. No matter how experienced I had become and how much I had worked with body and mind, I still kept a safe distance from the Kundalini energy. One day, a friend of mine told me that she had had an experience with her own Kundalini. She had allowed it to rise, and then it had decided to back down again into the sacrum. I was impressed by her courage and wondered if I would be able to muster the same. A few days later, I decided to see how far I could go. Forty years had gone by since that terrible week when I couldn't sleep. Again I sat down and focused on the Kundalini. There was a fear in me that I would revive the whole disastrous experience, like tilting over the fine construction that I called my life and that it had taken me so long to create with one whimsical attempt at being brave. When I looked down internally I could see the snake. It was wrapped around my hip and waved in front of my pubic bone with the head stretched somewhat out like a sensing organ. It was aware of my presence. I asked it to slowly rise into my head. Every time I felt fear, I asked it to slow down and it did. Finally, it reached up to merge with the crown chakra at the top of my skull. After letting it stay there for some time, I asked it to slowly return to the sacrum. Again it obeyed. When it curled up in the sacrum there was a sigh of relief in my body. I worried that I might not be able to sleep later that night. Then it dawned on me: the Kundalini was a friend. We were working together and had probably done so for a long time. There was nothing to be afraid of any longer.

When I look back at that young man, I see how much I have healed since those terrible things happened. I can also see all the benefits that he received, like the sensitivity that became his most important tool in writing and in working with clients, and the presence of Self that he was forced to cultivate. At the same time, I have a feeling that something was broken that will probably never be healed. I was a pretty normal guy who was forcefully bent out of shape. In my inner vision, the boy was always standing in the middle of the river of life, while I am high up at the brink of it, looking down, somehow prevented from entering it again. I don't know if it will ever happen.

I have written much more extensively about my Kundalini experience in the novel: *Darkness Without Limits*. Reprinted by Austin Macauley Publishers, 2024.

3

WHAT IS THE KUNDALINI?

Before we move on to discuss how to work with the Kundalini, I will describe what the Kundalini actually is—and also, in the next chapter, what IFS is—as this therapy creates the foundation of the way I work with the serpent energy.

In India, the concept of Kundalini has existed for thousands of years with roots deep into mysticism and philosophy. It is a central element of many religious disciplines and traditions in Hinduism, Buddhism, and Tantra. As such it is mentioned in many of the old religious texts. But the concept has also been taken up by modern spirituality and New Age movements, transforming it from a sacred, religious practice to personalized self-development.

In Eastern spirituality, there is no complete consensus about what Kundalini is and where it lives in the body. The main concept is that Kundalini is a primordial, spiritual source or life force in the shape of a serpent that resides dormant and coiled up at the bottom of the spine, in front of or inside the sacral bone, in the so-called root chakra. We are born with it, and it is aware of everything we are doing. The name Kundalini comes from Sanskrit and means coiled up or circular, hinting at the cyclical nature of this energy, connected to birth, life, death, rebirth, and stepping out of the karmic wheel.

The aim of these traditional texts is not to gain supernatural powers or participate in excesses of sensual pleasures, which sometimes seems to be the case in the modern use of Kundalini.

Kundalini is known as a divine energy and is used as a name for female goddesses, among them Shakti.

When it is awakened, it rises through the seven chakras or energy centers of the body, from the root chakra at the bottom of the spine, to the crown chakra at the top of the head. These chakras are in the religious belief imagined to be situated along the spine and are closely linked to the perception of the Kundalini. The chakras can be understood as different nerve plexuses—like the solar plexus. Symbolically they are pictured as lotuses or wheels with a varied number of petals or spokes.

Sometimes the Kundalini will awaken spontaneously, as was the case with me, but it normally happens through spiritual exercises like meditation, yoga, mantra chanting, tantric rituals, bandhas (energy locks), pranayamas (breathing exercises), and asanas (somatic exercises).

There are two ways of Kundalini awakening: one is active, the other is passive. The active way is forcing it to rise, as I've described above.

The passive way is about surrender, where one lets go of all that is blocking the awakening rather than trying to actively force the Kundalini to rise. An important part of this approach is what is known as *shaktipat,* which means the transmission of spiritual energy by a teacher or a guru. Fundamentally, it is a way to awaken the Kundalini by someone who already knows how to do this. Shaktipat only raises Kundalini temporarily, but it gives the student an experience of what is happening, which makes it much easier to process the fear.

The structure of this passive surrender is mirrored in the way IFS works, as it is a so-called *constraint release model.* It means that in IFS we assume that the person is inherently healthy, equipped with a non-destructible Self, and that what is needed in the therapeutic process is to let go of the constrictions that hinder health and the free expression of Self. Working with the constraints is an important part of the work with the Kundalini through IFS, and I'll come back to that in Chapter 4.

Under normal circumstances, it is not easy to awaken the Kundalini. It is a complex process that, according to tradition, demands discipline, dedication, and a guide to help navigate.

In preparation of integrating this spiritual energy, tradition teaches that a period of careful purification and strengthening of the body and nervous system is required. The body and the spirit must be prepared by the above-mentioned techniques and exercises. Then the Kundalini is ready to be awakened by a guru.

In the modern interpretation of Kundalini, the focus is not so much on the snake aspect itself, but more on perceiving it as a universal life energy that can be found in many places in the body. A spontaneous Kundalini awakening, however, is something else entirely. Perhaps it is best described as a consuming fire that runs up the spine and leaves only ashes. It is important to keep in mind that this destructive process is the topic of this book.

The different traditions do not agree on what happens during a Kundalini awakening. I will not be going into details about differences, but rather present a description based on how I, following my incident, was taught that the Kundalini rises.

When the Kundalini energy is being awakened, it starts to rise like a serpent up through the spine from the root chakra. According to the gurus, it is supposed to awaken all the chakras on the way. Each chakra is believed to represent different aspects of our lives, and activating them should lead to a spiritual awakening and self-realization.

Again, according to the gurus, there are two currents inside or outside the spinal column, one called *Pingala* and another called *Ida*, that are believed to correspond to the sympathetic nervous system. Between them is a hollow canal called *Sushumna* that runs through the spinal cord that is supposed to correspond to the parasympathetic nervous system. At the lower end of the Sushumna is what is known as the *Lotus of the Kundalini*. It is seen as a triangle, where the Kundalini is coiled up. This is called the root chakra. The traditions differ as to the physical location—whether this is the coccygeal or the sacral plexus.

As it awakens, the Kundalini tries to force its way through the Sushumna. From the coccygeal or the sacral plexus, it moves upward through the lumbar and the higher dorsal, cervical, and medullary plexuses and reaches the spiritual eye at the point between the eyebrows to finally arrive at the crown chakra, the so-called thousand-petaled lotus (*Sahasrara*), at the top of the head. In Hinduism, we are asked to perceive Kundalini as the goddess Shakti's symbolical unification with the god Shiva in a cosmic wedding. The person then should become engrossed in deep meditation and infinite bliss. When the Kundalini reaches the brain, the person in which the awakening is happening is supposed to become detached from his or her body and mind, and his or her soul to be set free.

The union at the top of the skull should be felt as a cool breeze over the head or in the palms of the hands.

Raising the Kundalini is also a way to turn the life force or sexual energy inwards, into what in psychological terms is known as sublimation.

During the awakening, the Kundalini is said to purify, energize, and enlighten our being. This should lead to a deep transformation on a physical, mental, and spiritual level, giving not only mental clarity, increased intuition, strong sensitivity, and more self-awareness, but also euphoria and energy and a feeling of unlimited love and unity with the universe. The Self steps forward, and our highest consciousness unfolds. When it reaches the crown chakra, the person is said to have achieved spiritual enlightenment, so-called *unio mystica*, nirvana, or samadhi. The person transcends and is free of the Karmic wheel.

Besides the spiritual expansion when the Kundalini awakens, it can also lead to healing, psychical as well as psychological by dismantling blockages and re-creating balance in the body and mind. In that way, it should be able to help us move past traumas and create a feeling of well-being and inner peace.

Some gurus warn that spontaneous or premature Kundalini awakenings without guidance will not lead to the desired goal of enlightenment. Instead, it can lead to self-deception and misuse of power. From a Western perspective, this is probably true, but we also must take into consideration that it is a belief created in a hierarchical society where the gurus might want to hold on to their power. That said, with my story as an example, it is obvious that some individuals may experience very uncanny physical and psychological symptoms.

To further complicate things, we actually talk about two kinds of Kundalini: a Kundalini that moves upward (*urdhva*) and is associated with expansion, and a Kundalini that moves downward (*adha*) and is associated with contraction.

This movement is probably what I experienced, when I lay awake in bed, unable to move, and the energy either went up or down in my body.

CARL GUSTAV JUNG

As this is a book about how to work with the Kundalini energy through IFS, it is worth noting that the Swiss psychiatrist and psychoanalyst Carl Gustav Jung had discovered Kundalini and built part of his psychological theory on it.

In 1932, in the Psychological Club in Zurich, Carl Gustav Jung held a seminar on Kundalini yoga that is now widely acknowledged as a milestone in the Western psychological understanding of Eastern religion and philosophy. Jung saw the Kundalini awakening as an important map or description of the symbolic transformations of inner experience. It provided him with a model for cultivating higher consciousness that led to the notion of individuation, one of his most famous contributions to psychology.

Jung was also very aware of the dangers of experimenting with the Kundalini and believed that

Westerners should refrain from working with chakras higher than the heart chakra, as the energy, when the Kundalini connected with the higher chakras, would dangerously overwhelm them. According to Jung, the concept of Kundalini had only one purpose for Westerners, to experience the unconscious through the symbols of the awakening of the serpent.

Jung also realized that strange symptoms in clients, psychological as well as somatic, in a few cases could be explained by the awakening of the Kundalini. What was normally perceived as a pathological state, could actually be understood as very meaningful symbolic processes, through which the clients became healthier.

Some researchers have noted the similarities between the outcome of Kundalini practices and the experiences of Wilhelm Reich and his students in bioenergetic therapy, where the body for example can start to vibrate, as it releases constraints. It was bioenergetic therapy that helped me reconnect with my body, and I will be forever grateful for that.

Studies of transpersonal psychology and near-death experiences can also be linked to the Kundalini. Researchers have found signs of motor, mental, sensory, and affective symptoms that they have associated with the awakening. Sometimes this is called the Kundalini syndrome.

In the 1970's, psychologists and psychiatrists began noticing, perhaps unsurprisingly, that the more popular Eastern spiritual practices become in the West—especially meditation—the more psychological problems tend to emerge in individuals engaged in these practices. It also seems to affect people who experience spontaneous awakenings, almost as if the field of awakenings has become more common—or because we now have a new vocabulary to describe these events.

What happens during a Kundalini awakening can in many ways be perceived as an acute psychotic episode. In some instances, it can no doubt be necessary to give antipsychotic medication to people who are struggling with Kundalini, or maybe even give them the safety of being in a mental institution. Luckily, the more widespread the knowledge of Kundalini becomes, the more psychologists, psychotherapists, and psychiatrists will learn about this complex process, and at least a few of them will be able to understand that it is not a psychotic episode, but a spiritual process. At the same time, it is still important to warn people against these reactions. What happens during an awakening of the Kundalini is even today far from understood by professionals working in the mental health field.

According to brain researchers, what we perceive as spiritual or religious experiences can be explained as reactions in the nervous system and the brain. MR scans show that the brain activity changes in people who meditate, pray, or are feeling connected on a spiritual level. In that sense, spirituality can be a resource, particularly in healing, that gives positive and motivational experiences. We do not know, however, how much of the effect is placebo.

4

WHAT IS IFS
(INTERNAL FAMILY SYSTEMS)?

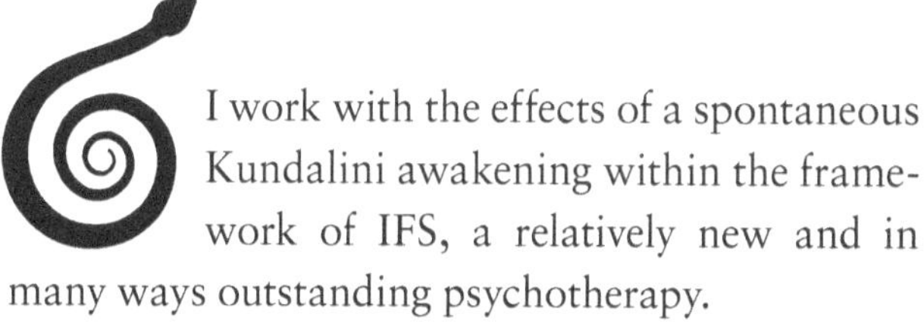

I work with the effects of a spontaneous Kundalini awakening within the framework of IFS, a relatively new and in many ways outstanding psychotherapy.

So what is IFS?

Internal Family Systems can best be described as an experimental, integrative, evidence-based, non-pathologizing psychotherapy, invented by the American Richard Schwartz and a cohort of people around him.

Richard Schwartz started as a young idealistic Family Therapist who wanted to *save the world*. Family Therapy is built on the assumption that if you help the members of a family to find their roles in relation to each other, the healing of the family will also happen in all of them. Richard Schwartz began a study of bulimic youth, mainly girls. Unfortunately, the result of the study didn't confirm what he had hoped. Family Therapy didn't appear to help the participants. From his father, a well-known medical scientist, he had learned to go with the data, even when it proved his thesis wrong. In a kind of desperation, Richard Schwartz began talking with the girls about what happened inside of them and noticed that they spoke about parts of them that did not want them to eat and other parts of them that did want them to eat. Richard Schwartz began interviewing these parts and discovered that they had their own agendas for the person they were living inside of, and that they could be very polarized.

One important breakthrough came while Richard Schwartz was working with a bulimic girl who was also a self-harmer cutting her wrists. In one long epic session, Schwartz tried to persuade the part to stop cutting the client, and finally, it agreed to do so.

At the next session, Richard Schwartz opened the door for the client and saw that instead of cutting the wrist of the client, the part had made a cut across her face, keeping the promise of not cutting her wrist.

At this point, Richard Schwartz simply gave up. He fell back in terror and said that the part had won and that he could not compete with it.

To his surprise, the part answered that it didn't want to win. When he asked what it wanted, it answered that it needed to get the client out of her body whenever she was being sexually abused and to control her anger, as it would otherwise force her into more abuse. This made a lot of sense. Richard Schwartz also got the impression that the part lived in the past and believed that the abuse was still going on.

From this incident, Richard Schwartz learned that no matter how negatively parts seem to behave, they always have a positive intention with what they are doing.

What, then, is IFS more specifically? Richard Schwartz claims that the psyche is multiple, that we consist of a lot of different parts, each with a separate identity and consciousness, and that they can work alone or in groups and hierarchies. Parts are not just feelings, sensations, or aspects of the psyche, but actual sub-personalities in us, each with their own feelings, agendas, and beliefs. Often they are polarized. In therapy, parts are important because they have access to implicit memory in ways that we do not. Parts are not only telling you what you already know, they actually contain a lot of information about things that you do not know, for instance about trauma, when and why it happened, and what impact it had on you.

Richard Schwartz brought the framework of systemic Family Therapy into his work with parts. Working systemically, he found that the psyche can be said to consist of three groups of parts that he called managers, firefighters, and exiles. Both managers and firefighters are parts of what is known as the protective system.

Managers are often the first parts we encounter, both when we meet people and when we work with clients in a clinical setting. They are proactive. From a societal point of view, managers are the good guys who make us behave well, in socially acceptable ways. They manage our lives, make us get up in the morning, go to work, take care of the kids, etc. Unfortunately, managers are also very rigid, with very fixed ways of perceiving things, and they can be quite cruel in their attempt to make the person in which they live look good in the eyes of society, like when they take the shape of the well-known inner critics to make the person conform. Managers were often created while the person was very young, and so we can in many cases consider them to be small kids that are now trying the best they can to take care of a grown-up's life. Two of their most important jobs are to keep the exiles with their pain under lock and to control the firefighters. One of the paradoxes related to managers is that they very often create the very situation they are trying to avoid. Their motto is: Never let it happen again!

Here are a few examples of managers:

- an intellectual, analyzing part
- an inner critic part
- a controlling part
- a distancing part
- a pleaser part
- a helper part
- a minimizer part
- an over-working part.

Firefighters are the second group of parts, and they also belong to the protective group, but they work in very different ways than the managers. The main concern of Firefighters is to get the person away from pain, and they shun no ways to do so. They are often not socially acceptable and are the parts of us that we want to go away or believe are "not me". They are very reactive and can step up within a split second if pain from the exiles emerges. They work in two ways, by numbing us or by making us escape. Like the managers, they are trying to keep the pain from the exiles away from the person's consciousness. They also react against the managers, whom they find much too strict. Firefighters have the ability to overrule the managers, and the managers hate them for it—with good reason, as it is often the managers who have to clean up the mess when a firefighter has taken over. Their motto is: When everything else fails!

Here are a few examples of firefighters:

- an angry part
- a shopping part
- a web surfer part
- a drinking part
- a drug-using part
- an unfaithful part
- a killer part
- a suicidal part.

The last group of parts are the exiles. They are the vulnerable and wounded parts of us, often small children, the ones who have experienced the full impact of trauma. They have been exiled from the system by the protectors and are desperate to break free of their exile and have their pain acknowledged and witnessed. This terrifies the protectors. They fear that the exiles will take over and make

the internal system unstable. You can't live with
that much pain exposed. Their motto is: Do not
forget me.

A few examples of exiles are:

- a part that feels that it is too much
- a part that feels that it is bad
- a part that believes that it is not good enough
- a part that believes that it is not worth anything
- a part that feels that it is not lovable.

In addition to the important discovery that
parts always have a positive intention, Richard
Schwartz also discovered that parts often do not
like their roles and are burdened with negative beliefs, misperceptions, and heavy emotional states.
Where parts in many other therapies are judged
at face value—the way you behave is bad—we see
in IFS the part and the burden as two separate
things—the burden is bad, but you are not a bad
part. When we help the parts to separate from the
burden, they are under normal circumstances very
interested in letting go of it. In IFS we can help
them do that.

As Richard Schwartz worked with the parts in his clients, they sometimes began talking about *a part that was not a part*. When it showed up, it seemed that the sessions began to go faster and deeper and that it became much easier for the clients to heal. They also called it the self—or the Self, as Schwartz writes it with a capital S, to emphasize its uniqueness and importance. As Richard Schwartz talked with the Self and got to know it better, he slowly realized that it was what we can call the divine part of ourselves, our soul, our spiritual core, who we really are. In that sense, we already have a lot of descriptions and names for the Self in religious literature, where it is called Spirit, Christ-consciousness, Atman/Brahman, Highest Being, Source, etc. A core belief in IFS—supported by what the Self tells us about itself—is that we all have a Self, even though it can be hidden behind parts to protect it, and that this Self cannot be destroyed.

Like the discovery that parts only have positive intentions and that parts are not their burdens, the discovery of the Self had a huge impact on IFS therapy.

Richard Schwartz found that the Self can be characterized by eight qualities that all start with a C:

1. compassion
2. curiosity
3. confidence
4. calmness
5. creativity
6. courage
7. connectedness
8. clarity.

Two of the most important C-qualities are compassion and curiosity. A crucial difference between parts and the Self is that parts have all kinds of agendas while the Self only has the agenda to connect and allow love to flow in the system. To be able to do that, the Self has to *unblend* from the parts.

Most of the work in IFS takes place between the Self and the client's parts, with the therapist as a kind of guide helping the client's internal process unfold without giving any advice or analysis, simply being open, asking relevant questions and holding the space.

In order to do so, the therapist must be able to work from the Self, without the ever-present agendas of the parts. To achieve this, the therapist is constantly working on him- or herself and being aware if he or she is blended with a part, especially during sessions.

Richard Schwartz discovered another thing that is crucial in working with the Kundalini—that *the inner world can't attack me if I'm not afraid of it*. I made that same discovery during my challenge with the snakes, where I discovered that they couldn't bite me when I offered my finger to them. I have also experienced it with inner vampires that want to suck blood from my jugular vein. When I expose my neck and the vein to them, they can't carry through with their intention. If I had known that my fear fueled the Kundalini in my awakening, my process would have been very different and much easier. If fearful parts turn up, we can listen to them and address their fear, and then ask them to step back or leave the room, so that we can be with the Kundalini from the calm quality of Self.

In an IFS session, the client normally sits with closed eyes and connects to the parts from Self. This technique we call in-sight. In instances where the parts in the client will not allow the client's Self to step forward, the therapist may have to address the parts in directly. This technique we call direct access. This is the technique I primarily use to work with the Kundalini.

In IFS, we work with two protocols, one called *The 6 F's* and the other *The Healing Steps*. The 6

F's are about connecting to the part of the client
that we work with and communicating with that
part and getting to know it, while The Healing
Steps are about the unburdening of the exiles and
the integration into the system. As the work with
Kundalini is not about unburdening it, but getting
to know it and talking with it, the focus is on The
6 F's.

THE UNBURDENED SYSTEM

When exiles, managers, and firefighters let go of
the burdens they carry, the client's system becomes
increasingly unburdened. The system will now begin to function in a new way where the parts are
not fighting each other and are not polarized. Instead, they start working together under the lead-
ership of the Self, which they grant the power to
do so. The parts do not function well without the
presence of the Self, and the Self needs the parts to
take action, feel feelings, get ideas—to exist in the
world.

Managers who are liberated from the responsibility of having to stir the person's life become kind
of highly trusted servants to the Self. They are no
longer reacting to what happened, trying to avoid
and mend the past, but have a realistic view of

what is going on and how to react in proper ways to the benefit of the system. And as the most important exiles are being healed, they do not have to worry that they will overflow the system with pain.

Firefighters can also start to relax because the pain from the exiles is gone and no longer posing a threat to the system. The much-misunderstood firefighters turn out to be very valuable parts of us, who like to relax and play and not work as much as the managers would like us to. They are creative, impulsive, and keen on guiding us to the joys of life.

The exiles, liberated from exile and no longer burdened by pain and false beliefs about themselves, can now become what they were meant to be: loving, playful, creative children who dare trusting others and enjoy creating connections.

The person will feel that a lot of high-strung drama has left his or her life, that there is calm and perspective, and that he or she can finally trust themselves. When the inner world is healed, we experience our relationships healing in the outer world. This will not make all problems in our life disappear, but we are now equipped with new-found resources and tools to deal with them. We can meet life from Self.

5

WORKING WITH THE KUNDALINI

WARNING: I cannot advise you to work with the Kundalini the way I present it here, especially if you don't have solid experience with IFS and in general know what you are doing in the therapy room. The first rule is not to do harm and to never bring a client to a place from where you can't bring him or her back again.

One day at my clinic, a client told me that she had some strange energy movements up and down her spine that made her afraid. It felt like a snake. She asked me if I could help her. Normally I would have asked her to lie down on my table so that I could get her to release the energy and the fear through the body, as it felt like the safest way. At the same time, I knew that this client was working intensely with a spiritual teacher and that she was very committed to what she called self-realization.

Working with IFS, you can decide to perceive anything as a part, even elements that initially do not present themselves as such. An example is burdens we try to help the parts to let go of in the unburdening process, which is a step in The Healing Steps protocol. When a part had difficulty in letting go of a burden, I discovered that I could talk directly to the burden and from its point of view learn why the release was so difficult. Normally we do not extend compassion or any other of the eight C-qualities of the Self to burdens, but I found that even burdens often hungered for love and understanding and for being heard. When I got them to understand that I could help them to free themselves from the part that they were attached to and that, in the process, they could transform the negative energy they consisted of into something positive or simply evaporate, they were always willing to let go of the attachment to the part. For the part, it was a relief to feel the burden leaving.

Here it is worth mentioning we can work with not only burdens as parts, but also elements, beings, and conditions as diverse as a landscapes, organs, internalized parents, ghosts, ancestors or cancers.

As I was sitting with the client, I was thinking along these lines and wondered what would happen if I asked for permission to speak to the serpent in her directly, as I had often done with the burdens. When I suggested this, she had enough faith in me to say yes.

In IFS, we know that we can ask parts to *turn down the volume*, to become less intense but stay connected to us if other parts of the system feel that there is a risk that these parts can overwhelm the client. I told her about this technique and that I would use it if the snake tried to take over. From my own experience, I knew what harm the Kundalini could cause, and my most important concern was to keep her safe and avoid any uncontrolled awakening of the Kundalini. I was prepared to shut down the session immediately if there was a risk that things got out of control.

Using direct access, I asked for permission to talk to the serpent. The client checked in with it, and it was surprised to be contacted but willing. I told it that it could use the client's voice so that we could speak together. I also told it that for this to work, it would have to refrain from overwhelming the client, which it agreed to, even though it told me that it was more than willing to help the client by rising to the top of her head.

During the next twenty minutes, I spoke with the snake. There were many times that I had to ask it to turn down the intensity because it became so eager. I told it that humans were unable to endure the strong energy that it carried if we didn't go slow, and it admitted being aware of that. It revealed that its purpose was to heal and enlighten the client. It wanted to show the client some secrets that it knew she was afraid to get to know. When I checked with the client, she admitted that there were spiritual fields that she didn't dare to enter from fear of what it would reveal and of never coming back.

The serpent also knew this. It assured her that it would always bring her back. It didn't want to harm her in any way, but its eagerness brought it into trouble.

After about twenty minutes, when we had received a lot of information, and the serpent slowly had been permitted to go through the spine, up into the head, and meet the crown chakra, where it rested, it said that it was tired, and wanted to go back into the sacrum.

This came as a total surprise to me. I had not expected that this strong energy would become tired. I thought of the relentless snake energy, pressing and pressing up into my head. Had I known at the time that there was a way of dealing with it, my life would have looked very different. For a moment I had a bitter taste in my mouth.

The serpent descended slowly through the spine and lay itself to rest in the sacrum. Then it fell asleep, tired as it was.

I checked how the client was doing, and we discussed the information that the serpent had given her. She felt ready to continue on her spiritual path. The fear was gone. I naturally checked in with her over the coming days, weeks, and months, but the Kundalini didn't cause her any more problems. It was present, but if it became too eager, she could always ask it to be less intense. It understood that if it wanted to help her, it had to adapt to her pace.

I wish I had known these techniques when I was 18 years old.

When I begin a session where I will be working with the Kundalini, I do it in the way it is normally done in an IFS session. I ask the client to go inward, close their eyes, and focus on the body. In a Kundalini session, I'm even more attentive to letting the client feel his or her body than in an ordinary session. I want to make sure that the client can sense the support of the body.

Then I ask the client if any parts have anything against us working with the Kundalini. This is an important step, as I want the client's Self to be *unblended* from parts before we move on. There will often be fearful parts that need to be heard. We can assure them that they are in control, and that they can close down the session any moment they feel it is no longer safe. We also tell these parts that they can sit by and watch the session from the sideline, and that, if needed, I have a lot of experience in asking the Kundalini to turn down the intensity. Normally this will make the parts relax. We stay here until all parts that have made themselves known are ready to move on.

From my Rolfing practice, I know that there are several *locks* in the body where it can contract, keeping feelings, memories, trauma, and energy from moving upwards. The legs have several of these locks, but what is interesting in this context are the ones in the torso. At the top of the sacrum is the first lock, traditionally the one that keeps the Kundalini encaged. Moving through the stomach area can be difficult for the serpent because we also can contract here, but I wouldn't consider it a definite lock. The diaphragm is a strong lock, and so is the shoulder area, entering the neck. The brainstem is capable of giving some resistance, but again, I would not consider it a real lock. However, it does help slow down the Kundalini before entering the skull, which is often one of the most scary and challenging moments for the client. From here there is free access to the crown chakra.

If I look at the locks through an IFS lens, they are areas in the body that are controlled by protector parts. This means that we can work with them in the same way as we normally work with parts. We can listen to their concerns and fears and address them, help them understand that they have to grant us access before we can move on, and that they can, at any moment, make the body contract again if they feel that what is happening is dangerous to the system. We build trust when we tell the parts that they are in control, and that we won't allow the Kundalini to overwhelm the system, which is what they are afraid of.

The Kundalini will often have moved somewhat up the spine already, for instance to the heart. To make sure that everything is fine, I often start by asking how the lock in the sacrum, which normally holds the Kundalini down, is doing. I may ask for permission to talk with it in direct access, to hear if it feels forced open, or if it is fine with the Kundalini having moved past it. If there is a problem, I will ask the lock if it would prefer, if I, a little later, when I speak with the serpent, call for it to come back down into the sacrum, so that we can start all over and do the unlocking together in a way that also feels right to the lock. I also ask the Kundalini the same question.

After this, I will normally ask the client where he or she can feel the Kundalini in the body. When we have identified it, most frequently from the position of its head, I check to see if my own Kundalini is present. As a general rule, it is, and if so, I ask the client's Kundalini if it is aware. Registering that I am familiar with working with this energy, it seems to calm it down. It starts to become more trustful.

I will also check if the Kundalini is aware of the client that it lives inside. Normally it is, but it can be necessary to allow it time to get to know the client better.

If it is necessary to do the unlocking of the sacrum, I would do that here.

Then we can start helping it ascend through the spine. I tell the serpent that we humans are unable to endure the strong energy that it embodies when pushing its way through. And I tell it that if it wants to achieve its goal of reaching the crown chakra, it needs to turn down the intensity. I will also ask if it has been successful in trying to push through, and it usually tells me no, so I offer to help it by doing it another way. The serpent understands this and will often admit that it knows that humans can't endure its energy. When I ask why it doesn't tone it down, it always answers that it is too eager, it wants to push through.

Again I check if all parts of the client are fine with what is happening. If not, we talk with them and address their concerns.

After the lock at the sacrum, the stomach area can be difficult for the serpent to get through, but if it does, it meets one of our strong protective muscles, the diaphragm. In my experience from working with Rolfing clients, the diaphragm can be considered the membrane between the unconscious and the conscious, and crossing it can be a challenge for some parts. Unless the serpent is going really slow, it won't be allowed to pass.

At the diaphragm, we check what parts are active towards the Kundalini and what their concerns and fears are. Can they be addressed? Most times the problem is that the Kundalini is moving too fast and is too eager. Then I talk with it and make it realize that going too fast has not worked for it yet, but that I can help it do it another way, by going very slow, by bringing the pace almost to a halt.

When the Kundalini has passed the diaphragm, I ask if it wants to continue directly to the head, or if it wants to connect with the heart first. Normally, it wants to meet the heart. I then ask the client if he or she is fine with that. If he or she says yes, we can help the Kundalini slowly branch off and move towards the heart. It normally wants to get its head inside the heart. This is the point where Carl Gustav Jung said Westerners shouldn't go higher, and indeed for some serpents, this seems to be enough for them. They like to be connected to the heart.

If the Kundalini wants to go higher, and the client agrees, I invite it to go back down into the spine and then slowly rise again. Maybe it needs to be reminded that it has to go slow, especially as it enters the neck, where we also have a strong lock.

The most critical place is the transition from the spine and medulla and into the cranium. I insist that we go slow here and are in constant communication with the client to hear if it is OK. Normally he or she will slowly allow the serpent's head to enter the cranial cavity. It is a good idea to pause when that has happened, and then when the serpent is ready finally let it rise to the crown chakra. It is happy to be allowed to do this.

The first few times I worked with the Kundalini this way, I was actually not sure if it was supposed to stay here. And I was surprised when the serpent suddenly told me that it was tired of standing so erect and that it wanted to retreat down the spine to relax in the sacrum. It made a lot of sense to me and it was a great relief, both to the client and me, that this strong force also could get tired. In my experience, it doesn't need to go back up again, although it can, if needed, for instance through tantric exercises, but the urgency and the eagerness is gone and because of this the client will no longer be afraid when the Kundalini wants to rise. The whole system can relax.

One element can be added to this "protocol". It is not common knowledge, but I have learned from the clients who come with a Kundalini awakening, that in the inner world, we have two big stones inside of us, often in or a little below the hip area. These stones may be hidden in dirt in that area and will have to be dug free. One stone, belonging to the right side of the hip and leg, is female. The other, belonging to the left side, is male and somewhat bigger than the female. Often they are very fond of each other. In clients who have not had a Kundalini experience, I have never encountered these stones, which could indicate that they are only awakened when there is a need for them.

Their task is to keep us connected to the ground and to prevent us from *flying away*. They move up and down in the body to help us remain in balance and adaptable to change. Like the Kundalini, they are very eager and can create pains when they want to go down the client's body too fast. They bring connectedness to the body and serve as a counter-balance to the uprising energy of the Kundalini. They bring safety.

An important question to consider is whether it is always safe to work this way with the Kundalini? My first answer is that the therapist should be able to be in what in IFS is called *Self-energy*. That means meeting the serpent from the Self. The therapist must also be sure to have professional skills and experience and importantly not be afraid of what happens in the inner world, both in the client and in him- or herself. IFS is not a resource-building modality. The modalities that strive to build resources in the client often give the reactive part, in this case, the Kundalini, the impression that it is not wanted in the system, for instance by asking the client to ground or to breathe in a certain pattern to suppress it. In IFS, we go directly to the reactive part, inviting it to be present, and asking what made it so reactive? We build trust by acknowledging and connecting with the part, and the information it gives us helps us understand what it requires to be able to relax. Contrary to what one might think, the more reactive the part is, the more it needs to be met this way. In my experience, this also applies to working with the Kundalini. The more desperate it is to rise to the crown chakra, the more it needs our help. And so does the client.

The pitfalls in this process are being afraid of what is happening and not going slow enough. It's important for the therapist to have sufficient authority or Self-energy to ask the serpent to slow down and dial down the intensity in a convincing way. As always in therapeutic work, it is crucial to have strict boundaries and be able to help the client take over the responsibility of the process when he or she is ready.

In the days after working with the Kundalini, it is a good idea to check in with the client and to discuss the experience during the next session to see if a follow-up is needed. I always let the process run until the Kundalini by itself declares that it is tired and wants to return to the sacrum. Doing that seems to prevent any backlashes. Finally, the work with the stones can also bring more balance and "weight" to the system.

6

A SESSION

The following is a session I had with a client, Karen, who came to me because the Kundalini energy caused her discomfort, anxiety, and problems with sleeping. Karen was 58 years old, heterosexual, divorced, had two grown-up kids and worked as an interior designer. I had been working with her for several years. The problem had started after she had been on a several-week-long spiritual retreat. She had some disturbing visions of snakes in her spine and was afraid that she was going mad.

I suggested that I could try to talk with the snake, and she eagerly agreed to that.

Me: Try to focus on the serpent. Where do you feel it in or around your body?

Karen: I feel it here. (She was pointing to her upper stomach area). A bit higher than the navel button.

Me: Is it OK if I try to speak to it?

Karen: Yes.

Me: Serpent in the upper part of Karen's stomach, are you there?

(There was a pause).

Serpent: Yes.

Me: Thank you for speaking to me. Is it OK if I try to get to know you a little bit better?

Serpent: Yes.

Me: What is happening right now?

Serpent: I'm stuck here.

Me:　　Are you stuck inside the spine?

Serpent:　　Yes. I can't move back or forward. She is squeezing my head.

Me:　　Some parts of her probably got scared. Sometimes you serpents are a bit too intense for us humans and then we close down. Will you be willing to let me help you?

Serpent:　　Yes. I want to get out.

Me:　　First of all I have to ask you to not be so intense. Will you be willing to turn down the volume? I'm not saying that you should shut down totally, just that you need to bring your energy down to a level where Karen can tolerate it. If you do that, I'll be able to help you. Are you willing to do that?

Serpent:　　Yes.

Me:　　OK. Does that give you a little more wiggle room?

Serpent: Yes. I'm so eager to get up into her head. I can't wait.

Me: Remember what I said. You have to slow down, not be too intense. Karen will be afraid and then you'll just get stuck again.

(The serpent doesn't answer, and I take that as a sign that it agrees).

Me: Are you aware of Karen, that you live inside of her?

Serpent: Yes.

Me: Do you know who she is?

Serpent: Yes, she is the grown-up with the light inside of her.

Me: That is right. Is she someone you feel that you can trust?

Serpent: Yes. I want to help her, but she won't allow me.

Me: That is because you go too fast. We
                 need to slow down. What is it that
                 you want to help Karen with?

Serpent: There is a place that she wants to go.
                 I can help her with that.

Me: What kind of place is that?

Serpent: This is the place where all the mas-
                 ters are.

Me: So you can help her with meeting the
                 spiritual masters?

Serpent: Yes. And the spiritual energies. But
                 she is afraid.

Me: What is she afraid of?

Serpent: She is not sure what will happen af-
                 terward. She believes that she has to
                 stay there.

Me: So she is afraid that she will not be
                 able to come back to a normal life. Is
                 that a concern?

Serpent: No. I'll help her back.

Me: Karen, did you hear what the snake said?

Karen: Yes.

Me: How do you want to respond to that?

Karen: It is true that I have that fear, but I also think that deep down, I know that I will be able to come back. Nevertheless, it is comforting to hear the serpent say that.

Serpent: (addressing me): It's a beautiful serpent you have. I like it.

Me: Thank you. I'm sure it is curious to see who you are.

(We sit a moment in silence, and I sense how the client's and my serpent are acknowledging each other with a slight wave of their heads and upper bodies, like two cobras).

Me: Is it OK if I get curious about who you are?

Serpent: Yes. What do you want to know?

Me: I have never been totally clear on whether you are a life force or sexual energy.

Serpent: That is a weird question that I can't answer.

Me: Why not?

Serpent: Because I'm both. You can't separate that.

Me: Thank you for enlightening me on this. That is important for me to know. Where do you come from? Are you ancient, or do you only live inside of Karen?

Serpent: I'm ancient. And I come from deep down.

Me: Deep down inside of us or?

Serpent: Inside and outside. I'm both. I come
               from the deep caves.

Me: So you are very primordial?

Serpent: Yes, I was here from the beginning.

Me: And are you different serpents in
               each of us humans, or are you the
               same serpent in all of us?

Serpent: I'm both. We are in all humans, but
               we come from the same source. We
               are one.

Me: Thank you for telling me that. If
               I should help you to get out of that
               stuck place you are in, would you
               first like to go down into the sacrum
               and start all over again?

Serpent: No. I'm so eager to get up into her
               head.

Me: I'll just check with the parts that held
               the sacrum locked and hear what
               they have to say. Parts, are you there?

Lock-parts: Yes.

Me: How do you feel about letting the serpent rise through the spine, if we do it slowly? I'll not let the serpent take over. You can stand by and be ready to step in if you feel that things are going too fast.

Lock-parts: It's OK.

Me: Will you be ready to let the channel be open?

Lock-parts: Yes.

Me: Are there any parts at the diaphragm that have concerns about letting the snake through?

Karen: I can feel one or two scared parts.

Me: What are they afraid will happen?

Karen: They fear that the energy will overwhelm the system and… and that I
might die.

Me: What if we told those parts that we
will go very slow and that I can ask
the serpent to dial down the volume
if it gets too strong—how do they
feel about that? They have the power, they can stop the process anytime
they want.

Karen: They are cautious but willing to step
to the side. They'll be very attentive.

Me: That is great. Just ask them to stand
by and watch what is happening.
They can always step in.

Me: Serpent, are you ready to slowly move
through the diaphragm?

Serpent: Yes, I almost can't hold back.

Me: You have to. You have to slow down. You know what happens if you push forward. Then you'll just get stuck. Go really slow, don't be too intense.

Serpent: OK. But it is hard. But I see what you mean.

(The serpent moves through the diaphragm).

Me: Is it OK, Karen?

Karen: Yes. But I'm almost at my limit.

Me: Serpent, go slow. Then you'll get there.

(The head of the serpent comes into the chest).

Me: Do you want to go to the heart or move upwards to the head?

Serpent: (considering for a while): To the heart.

Me: Then wait here. I'll check with Kar-
            en if that is OK. Karen, you heard
            the serpent. Is it OK if it goes to the
            heart first?

Karen: Yes, if it goes slow.

            (The serpent slowly slides into the
            heart with the head. It stays there for
            a while).

Me: How does it feel, Karen?

Karen: Actually good. Like a new connec-
            tion is being made.

Me: Serpent, will it be OK to move on?

Serpent: Yes.

Me: Do you want to go back into the sa-
            crum or go to the head?

Serpent: I want to go to the head!

Me: We have to go slowly. Is it OK with
            you, Karen?

Karen: Yes.

(When the serpent gets closer to Karen's neck, I can see that she starts to become anxious and breathe more rapidly. Her eyelids are flickering).

Me: Is it going too fast?

Karen: Yes.

Me: Serpent, you have to slow down and turn down the intensity.

Serpent: I just want to get into the head.

Me: I can help you with that, but if you don't do it slowly, you'll get stuck again.

(The serpent slows down).

Me: Is it OK now?

Karen: Yes.

Me: Serpent, when you start to get into the skull you have to move really slow. It can be very scary for us humans. Just allow your snout to come in and let us see how Karen feels.

Karen: Actually it is OK because it is moving so slowly. It feels respectful.

(The serpent comes into the skull and starts to move to the crown chakra. When it reaches that, a calm spreads in Karen's system).

Me: How does it feel now?

Karen: It actually feels really good now. There is no more push.

(The serpent stays connected to the crown chakra for some time).

Serpent: Now I'm tired. I want to go down.

Me: How was it for you to be connected?

Serpent: Great, but now I want to go down.

                (It quickly slides backward into the sacrum).

Karen: I think it fell asleep.

Me: That is also what I see. It must have been tired. We can just let it rest there. This may sound weird, but can you see a stone in your hip?

Karen: No.

Me: Is it OK if I try to speak to it directly?

Karen: Yes.

Me: Can I speak with the stone that is in Karen's hip?

Stone: Yes, who are you?

Me: I'm helping Karen to relate better to the serpent, and I would like your help in doing that.

Karen: Now I can see it. It is weird. It is a female stone.

Me: Let it know that you are there.

Karen: It has become very heavy now, giving me a lot of pain.

Me: Stone, you are pressing too hard. Can you ease up somewhat?

Stone: That is true. You humans are so fragile. Where is my companion?

Me: You mean the other stone?

Stone: Yes. I can't see it.

Me: Maybe it is buried.

Stone: Oh, yes, here it is.

Me: Karen, can you help the stone to dig the dirt away from the other stone?

Karen: Yes, it was totally covered, but now I see it. It is a male stone. They seem to be partners.

Me: Stone, what are you doing for Karen?

Stone: We keep her balanced.

Me: Balancing, how? So that she won't fly away from too much energy?

Stone: Yes, we make her heavy, but it is all a question about balance.

Me: Great. How do you do that?

Stone: We go down into her legs.

Me: That sounds really good. Is there more you would like to let us know?

Stone: Not right now.

Me: How do you feel, Karen?

Karen: Light and heavy and very relaxed. There is no fear.

Me: Would it be OK to stop the session
             here and come back to the outer
             world?

Karen: Yes.

END

After having worked with my clients with Kundalini issues and having my own initial experience with it, I no longer believe that the right way to connect with the Kundalini is by trying to force it to rise from the sacrum with meditation, exercises, controlled breathing, etc. I do not believe in the wisdom of these old, religious practices. It seems to be a way to make the Kundalini and the body do something that they do not want to do, like when poking and irritating a snake with a stick, especially when the Kundalini still hasn't awakened. When it has awakened and wants to go to the crown chakra, the body will often perceive it as an internal violation and create a host of negative reactions. The process might have a noble purpose, the achievement of wisdom and enlightenment, but as far as I can tell, it is still an exploitation with the use of external stressors,

especially since we now have the protocol present-
ed in this book for exploring the serpent energy.
Ideally, the awakening of the Kundalini should be
experienced as a gentle, natural process, where it
rises and then falls on its own volition—like the
ebb and flow of the sea. The Kundalini should vol-
untarily give us the gifts that it wants to. The way I
see it, the snake is much happier and feels respected
when it is welcomed like that.

SOURCES

Jung, C. G.: The Psychology of Kundalini Yoga – Notes of the Seminar Given in 1932. Princeton University Press, 1999. 128 p.

Legård Nielsen, Peter: Alle dele er velkomne: Internal Family Systems i teori og praksis. Forlaget Blå, 2024. 353 p.

Legård Nielsen, Peter: Darkness Without Limits. Reprinted by Austin Macauley Publishers, 2024. 187 p.

Odier, Daniel: Yoga Spandakarika: the sacred texts at the origins of Tantra. Inner Traditions, 2024. 1st ebook edition.

Saraswati, Satyananda: Kundalini Tantra. Yoga Publications Trust, 2016. 453 p.

Schwartz, Richard C. and Sweezy, Martha: Internal Family Systems Therapy. Second Edition. The Guilford Press, 2020. 304 p.

Yesudian, Selvarajan: Yoga uge for uge. Øvelser og meditationer til hele året. Thanning & Appel, 1977. 237 p.

www.ingramcontent.com/pod-product-compliance
Lightning Source LLC
LaVergne TN
LVHW051451170726
843492LV00002B/647
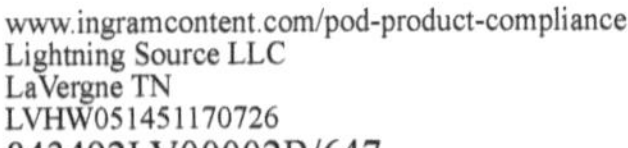